DASH DIET COOKBOOK FOR ALZHEIMER

Wholesome Flavors for Mindful Living and Brain Booster Meal for Alzheimer

Maria H. Tee

Copyright © 2023 Maria H. Tee

This book is a work of non-fiction. The views expressed are solely those of the author and do not necessarily reflect the publisher's view, and the publisher hereby disclaims any responsibility for them.

TABLE OF CONTENTS

INTRODUCTION

In the quiet town of Crestwood, there lived an elderly man named Samuel. Samuel had been grappling with the challenges of Alzheimer's disease, facing the gradual erosion of his memories and cognitive abilities. His family, particularly his devoted granddaughter, Emma, witnessed the toll the condition took on Samuel's once vibrant spirit.

Determined to make a difference, Emma delved into research on how nutrition could potentially support cognitive health. She discovered the concept of brain-boosting foods, particularly those aligned with the principles of the Dietary Approaches to Stop Hypertension (DASH) diet.

Emma, a passionate cook, decided to embark on a culinary journey to create meals that not only satisfied Samuel's palate but also nourished his brain. Armed with a plethora of colorful fruits, vegetables, lean proteins, and whole grains, Emma set out to transform her grandfather's diet.

She began with Samuel's favorite meal—breakfast. Instead of the usual pastries, she introduced him to blueberry and walnut overnight oats, explaining the benefits of antioxidants and omega-3 fatty acids for cognitive function. Samuel intrigued and appreciative of the delicious change, eagerly embraced this new morning ritual.

For lunch, Emma crafted a quinoa and chickpea salad, rich in proteins and packed with nutrients known to support brain health. Samuel, who initially had reservations about this unfamiliar dish, found himself savoring the diverse flavors and textures that danced on his taste buds.

Dinner became an adventure in culinary exploration. Emma prepared a baked cod with lemon and herbs, highlighting the importance of omega-3 fatty acids found in fish for maintaining cognitive well-being. Accompanying this dish was a hearty sweet potato and chickpea stew, designed to provide a wholesome and satisfying dinner.

As the weeks passed, Samuel's palate expanded, and so did the sparkle in his eyes. Emma noticed subtle improvements in his clarity of thought and memory recall.

Encouraged by these positive changes, she continued to experiment with brain-boosting recipes, tailoring them to Samuel's preferences and nutritional needs.

The impact of this dietary transformation extended beyond the kitchen. Samuel, once withdrawn and frustrated by his cognitive challenges, found a renewed sense of engagement with the world around him. He started to share stories from his past, recounting memories that had long been obscured by the fog of Alzheimer's.

Emma's commitment to integrating brain-boosting foods into Samuel's diet became a beacon of hope for their family. While Alzheimer's remained a part of their lives, the power of thoughtful and nutritious cooking had, in Samuel's case, become a source of resilience, connection, and moments of clarity amid the challenging journey.

In this small town, Samuel's story became a testament to the transformative potential of combining love, care, and brain-boosting nutrition in the fight against Alzheimer's disease. Alzheimer's disease is a progressive neurodegenerative disorder that primarily affects the brain, leading to a gradual decline in memory, cognitive function, and the ability to perform everyday activities.

It is the most typical cause of dementia, a word used to describe a mental deterioration severe enough to cause problems in day-to-day functioning.

Key features of Alzheimer's disease include the accumulation of abnormal protein deposits, such as beta-amyloid plaques and tau tangles, in the brain. These deposits disrupt communication between nerve cells and eventually lead to the death of brain cells.

The symptoms of Alzheimer's disease typically develop slowly and worsen over time. Early signs may include difficulty remembering recent events, challenges with problem-solving, confusion about time and place, and changes in mood or personality. As the disease progresses, individuals may experience difficulty speaking, swallowing, and performing basic tasks.

While the exact cause of Alzheimer's disease is not fully understood, it is believed to result from a combination of genetic, environmental, and lifestyle factors. Age is a significant risk factor and the prevalence of Alzheimer's increases with advancing age.

Some treatments and interventions can help manage symptoms and improve the quality of life for individuals and their caregivers. Ongoing research aims to better understand the mechanisms of the disease and develop new therapeutic approaches.

Alzheimer's has a significant impact not only on those diagnosed but also on their families, friends, and caregivers. Supportive care, education, and resources are essential for those affected by this challenging condition just like Samuel, early diagnosis and intervention can provide opportunities for individuals to receive appropriate care and help improvement.

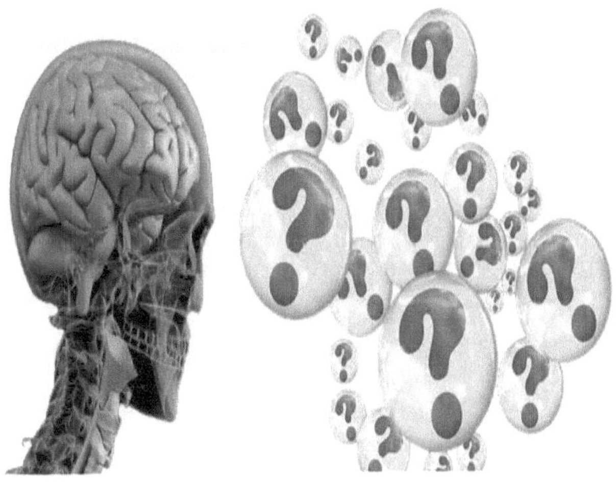

CHAPTER 1

Understanding Alzheimer's Disease and the Benefits of a Brain-Boosting Diet

Alzheimer's disease, a progressive neurodegenerative disorder, poses significant challenges for individuals and their loved ones. As we delve into the complexities of this condition, exploring avenues to support cognitive health becomes paramount. One promising approach is the adoption of a brain-boosting diet, tailored to nourish both the body and mind.

The Landscape of Alzheimer's Disease

Alzheimer's is characterized by the accumulation of abnormal protein deposits in the brain, disrupting neural communication and leading to cognitive decline. Symptoms, starting with mild memory loss, gradually progress to severe impairment, affecting daily activities.

Research indicates a strong link between diet and cognitive function. A brain-boosting diet focuses on nutrients that support brain health, including antioxidants, omega-3 fatty acids, vitamins, and minerals.

Proper nutrition may help mitigate the impact of Alzheimer's and support overall well-being.

Key Components of a Brain-Boosting Diet

1. Omega-3 Fatty Acids: Found in fish, flaxseeds, and walnuts, omega-3s contribute to brain structure and function, potentially reducing the risk of cognitive decline.

2. Antioxidant-Rich Foods: Berries, leafy greens, and colorful vegetables are rich in antioxidants, protecting the brain from oxidative stress associated with aging.

3. Whole Grains: Whole grains provide a steady supply of glucose, the brain's primary energy source, promoting sustained cognitive function.

4. Lean Proteins: Fish, poultry, and plant-based proteins support neurotransmitter production, aiding in communication between brain cells.

5. Vitamins and Minerals: Adequate intake of B-vitamins, vitamin E, and minerals like zinc and magnesium supports various cognitive functions.

The Benefits of a Brain-Boosting Diet for Alzheimer

1. Cognitive Support: Nutrient-dense foods contribute to optimal brain function, potentially slowing cognitive decline.

2. Mood Enhancement: Certain foods, like fatty fish and nuts, contain compounds linked to improved mood and reduced risk of depression.

3. Energy and Vitality: A well-balanced diet provides sustained energy, combating fatigue and supporting overall vitality.

4. Heart Health: Many brain-boosting foods also promote cardiovascular health, reducing the risk of conditions that may exacerbate Alzheimer's symptoms.

Implementing a Brain-Boosting Diet

Consulting with healthcare professionals, including nutritionists and physicians, is essential when implementing dietary changes for Alzheimer's patients.

Tailoring the diet to individual preferences, considering chewing and swallowing abilities, and fostering a positive dining environment contribute to successful dietary interventions.

Exploring the causes of Alzheimer's Disease

Alzheimer's disease, a progressive and devastating neurological disorder, affects millions of individuals globally. While the exact cause of this complex disease remains elusive, decades of research have provided valuable insights into the intricate interplay of various factors that contribute to its development.

Genetics, age, and lifestyle are among the primary factors that scientists believe play a role in the development of Alzheimer's disease. The most significant risk factor is advancing age, with the likelihood of developing Alzheimer's increasing exponentially after the age of 65.

Additionally, a family history of the disease can significantly elevate an individual's risk, suggesting a genetic component that predisposes certain individuals to Alzheimer's.

Researchers have identified specific gene mutations associated with familial or early-onset Alzheimer's, which represents a small percentage of cases. These mutations involve proteins such as amyloid precursor protein (APP), presenilin 1 (PSEN1), and presenilin 2 (PSEN2) that are involved in the production and clearance of amyloid-beta, a hallmark protein in Alzheimer's pathology.

In these familial cases, the inheritance of these mutated genes from one or both parents dramatically increases the risk of developing the disease. However, genetics alone cannot fully account for the prevalence of Alzheimer's disease, as the majority of cases are not directly linked to genetic factors.

Environmental factors, such as lifestyle choices and overall health, are believed to have a significant impact on the development of Alzheimer's disease.

Chronic conditions like cardiovascular disease, diabetes, and obesity have been linked to an increased risk of developing Alzheimer's. Additionally, factors such as high blood pressure, high cholesterol, and smoking have been identified as potential contributors to the disease.

Moreover, researchers have identified a correlation between cognitive engagement and the risk of Alzheimer's disease. Individuals who engage in mentally stimulating activities, such as reading, learning new skills, and engaging in social interactions, may have a lower risk of developing the disease. This suggests that maintaining an active and cognitively stimulating lifestyle may help to preserve brain health and potentially reduce the risk of Alzheimer's.

While the exact causes of Alzheimer's disease remain a subject of ongoing research and debate, it is clear that a multifaceted combination of genetic, age-related, vascular health and environmental factors contribute to its development.

Diagnosing Alzheimer

Diagnosing Alzheimer's disease is a complex and lengthy process that requires the expertise of medical professionals specialized in neurology and geriatric medicine. It involves a combination of assessments, medical tests, and exclusion of other possible conditions that can cause similar symptoms.

1. Medical History and Physical Examination: The process typically begins with a detailed medical history interview with the patient and their family members. The doctor asks questions about the symptoms, their duration, and any other relevant medical conditions. A comprehensive physical examination is also conducted to rule out other potential causes of cognitive decline.

2. Cognitive and Memory Testing: A series of cognitive tests are performed to assess memory, thinking abilities, language skills, attention span, problem-solving skills, and orientation. These tests help identify any significant decline in cognitive function.

3. Brain Imaging: Neuroimaging techniques, such as magnetic resonance imaging (MRI) or computed tomography (CT) scans, may be used to examine the brain structure and rule out other possible causes for cognitive decline, such as brain tumors or strokes. These imaging techniques can detect any visible abnormalities in the brain, such as shrinkage or the presence of amyloid plaques and neurofibrillary tangles, which are characteristic of Alzheimer's disease.

4. Neuropsychological Evaluation: A comprehensive assessment conducted by a neuropsychologist helps evaluate the patient's cognitive function in more detail.

5. Spinal Fluid Analysis: In some cases, a lumbar puncture, also known as a spinal tap, may be performed to obtain a sample of cerebrospinal fluid (CSF) for analysis. CSF is examined for the presence of biomarkers associated with Alzheimer's disease, such as amyloid beta and tau proteins.

7. Follow-up Assessments: Diagnosing Alzheimer's disease is not always straightforward, and in some cases, it requires multiple assessments over time to confirm the diagnosis.

Follow-up evaluations may be scheduled a few months or even years later to track the progression of symptoms and rule out other possible causes.

It is important to acknowledge that diagnosing Alzheimer's disease can be challenging, as many of its symptoms, such as memory loss and cognitive decline, can be seen in other conditions as well. Thus, a thorough evaluation by qualified professionals is critical to reach an accurate diagnosis.

CHAPTER 2

Nutrition and Diets for Alzheimer

Proper nutrition and diet play a crucial role in the management and overall well-being of individuals with Alzheimer's disease. As the disease progresses, individuals may experience changes in appetite, difficulty with eating, and challenges in maintaining a balanced diet. Therefore, it is important to focus on providing a nutritionally dense and easily manageable diet that supports brain health and overall physical well-being.

Consumption of nutrient-dense foods that are rich in vitamins, minerals, and antioxidants. This includes vegetables, fruits, whole grains, lean proteins (such as fish, poultry, and legumes), and healthy fats (such as olive oil and avocados). These foods provide essential nutrients for brain health and help maintain overall vitality.

Food that are high in omega-3 fatty acids, such as fatty fish (salmon, mackerel, and sardines), flaxseeds, and walnuts.

Omega-3 fatty acids have been shown to support brain health and reduce inflammation, potentially benefiting individuals with Alzheimer's disease.

Regular and adequate fluid intake prevents dehydration. Proper hydration is essential for maintaining cognitive function and overall health. Offer water, herbal teas, and fruit-infused water to increase fluid intake.

As the disease progresses, individuals may experience difficulty with chewing and swallowing. Modify the texture of foods as needed, such as pureeing or softening foods to make them easier to eat. Use dietitian-recommended strategies to ensure individuals receive proper nutrition while maintaining safety during mealtime and include familiar foods that the individual enjoys and is accustomed to. A sense of familiarity can help stimulate appetite and make mealtime more enjoyable.

Limit the consumption of processed foods, sugary snacks, and sugary beverages. These foods can contribute to inflammation and may negatively impact overall health. Whenever feasible, choose whole, unprocessed foods instead.

Seeking guidance from a registered dietitian with expertise in Alzheimer's and dementia nutrition can be highly beneficial. They can create personalized meal plans, address specific dietary needs, and provide recommendations on supplements, if necessary and they can help provide Support and assistance as individuals with Alzheimer's disease may require assistance and support during mealtime.

Ensure a calm and relaxed environment, offer assistance with utensils, and provide verbal cues to guide them through the eating process. Patience, understanding, and empathy are crucial when supporting individuals with Alzheimer's disease in their nutritional needs.

Remember, nutrition and diet play a significant role in promoting overall health and well-being for individuals with Alzheimer's disease.

Exercises for Alzheimer

Physical exercise has been shown to have various benefits for individuals with Alzheimer's disease. Regular exercise can help improve cognitive function, mood, sleep quality, and overall physical health.

Walking is a simple and low-impact activity that can be easily incorporated into daily routines. Encourage regular walks in a safe and familiar environment, such as a neighborhood or park. Walking can help improve cardiovascular health, mobility, and overall well-being.

For individuals with limited mobility or who may require additional support, chair exercises can be effective. These exercises typically involve seated movements that can help improve strength, flexibility, and circulation. Examples include seated leg raises, arm circles, and stretching exercises.

Dancing is a fun and engaging form of exercise that can stimulate both physical and cognitive abilities. Choose music that the individual enjoys and encourage simple dance movements, such as gentle swaying or tapping feet. Dancing can enhance coordination, balance, and social engagement.

Water aerobics or swimming in a pool can provide a low-impact and safe exercise option for individuals with Alzheimer's.

Water exercises can help improve strength, flexibility, and cardiovascular health. Ensure supervision and assistance if needed, and consider flotation aids or pool noodles for added support.

Cycling, either on a regular bicycle or a stationary bike, can be a beneficial form of exercise. It helps improve cardiovascular health, leg strength, and overall endurance. Depending on the individual's abilities, adjust the intensity, duration, and resistance levels to suit their needs.

Incorporating simple ball games, such as tossing or catching a soft ball, can help improve hand-eye coordination, motor skills, and encourage social interaction. Adapt the game to the individual's capabilities, ensuring safety and enjoyment.

It is essential to consult with a healthcare professional or a qualified exercise specialist, such as a physical therapist, to determine the most appropriate exercises for individuals with Alzheimer's disease. They can provide personalized recommendations based on the individual's abilities, safety considerations, and specific needs.

It is also important to consider any physical limitations, adapt exercises as necessary, and prioritize safety throughout the exercise routine.

Managing Stress for Alzheimer

Managing stress is essential for individuals with Alzheimer's disease as stress can exacerbate symptoms and impact overall well-being.

Create a peaceful and soothing environment for the individual. Minimize noise, distractions, and excessive stimulation. Maintain a consistent daily routine and provide a predictable schedule, as familiarity can help reduce anxiety and stress.

Also encourage engagement in familiar and enjoyable activities that promote a sense of purpose and accomplishment. These activities could include light exercise, listening to music, doing puzzles, or engaging in hobbies. However, it is important to adapt activities to the person's abilities and preferences as the disease progresses.

Introduce relaxation techniques that can help reduce stress and anxiety. These may include deep breathing exercises, gentle stretching, guided imagery, or meditation.

Encourage participation in simple relaxation activities that the individual can comfortably engage in.

Offer emotional support and reassurance to alleviate stress. Maintain a calm and patient demeanor when interacting with the person. Use comforting gestures, verbal cues, and positive reinforcement to promote a sense of security and well-being.

Encourage social interactions and maintain social connections with family members, friends, and support groups. Social engagement can help reduce feelings of isolation and provide emotional support. Organize regular visits or virtual meetings with loved ones to foster a sense of belonging and reduce stress.

Promote Physical Health: Physical health is closely linked to emotional well-being. Encourage regular exercise within the individual's capabilities. Physical activities, such as gentle walks or seated exercises, can help reduce stress, improve mood, and enhance overall health.

Maintain a Balanced Diet: Proper nutrition is essential for managing stress.

Ensure the person with Alzheimer's disease is receiving a well-balanced diet that includes a variety of nutrient-rich foods. Limiting caffeine and sugar intake may also help in managing stress levels.

Remember, managing stress for individuals with Alzheimer's disease requires a personalized approach. It is crucial to adapt strategies based on the individual's preferences, abilities, and stage of the disease. Regular communication with healthcare professionals, including doctors and Alzheimer's specialists, can provide additional guidance and support in managing stress effectively.

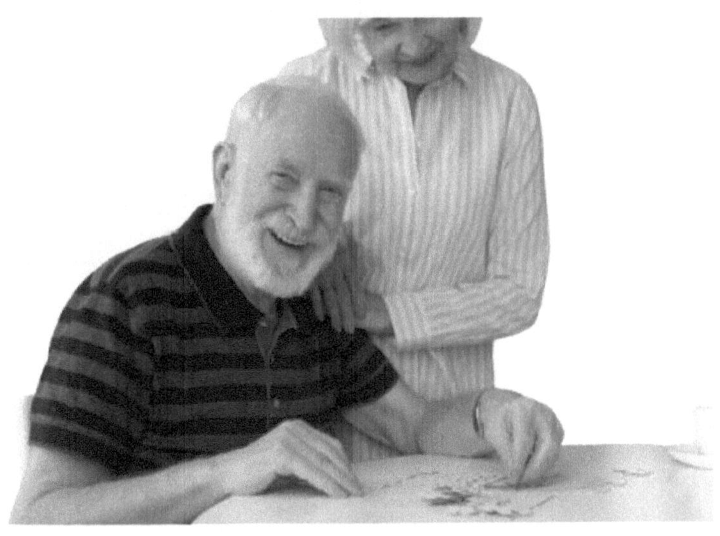

CHAPTER 3

Natural Therapies for Alzheimer

In the realm of Alzheimer's disease management, the integration of natural therapies stands as a compelling avenue, offering holistic approaches that address not only the symptoms but also the overall well-being of individuals navigating this challenging journey.

Engaging individuals with Alzheimer's in nature-based activities holds immense therapeutic value. Walks in natural settings, gardening, or birdwatching not only provide sensory stimulation but also foster a sense of connection with the environment, enhancing mood and cognitive engagement.

Aromatherapy, harnessing the aromatic essence of plant-derived essential oils, can have a calming and uplifting impact. Certain scents, such as lavender and rosemary, are believed to promote relaxation and may assist in managing symptoms of anxiety and agitation in Alzheimer's patients.

Certain herbal supplements are explored for their potential cognitive benefits. Ginkgo biloba, derived from the leaves of the ginkgo tree, is thought to improve blood flow to the brain. However, it's crucial to consult healthcare professionals before incorporating herbal supplements, as interactions with medications may occur.

Mindfulness practices, including meditation and guided imagery, contribute to stress reduction and enhanced emotional well-being. These techniques empower individuals with Alzheimer's to connect with the present moment, fostering a sense of tranquility and promoting mental resilience.

Integrating nutrient-dense superfoods into the diet may offer additional support. Food rich in antioxidants, such as blueberries, dark leafy greens, and turmeric, are believed to have anti-inflammatory properties that may benefit cognitive health.

Exposure to natural light, or light therapy, may positively impact sleep patterns and circadian rhythms, addressing issues commonly observed in Alzheimer's patients.

Access to natural daylight or specialized light boxes can be considered under the guidance of healthcare professionals.

Interactions with animals, whether through pet ownership or organized animal-assisted therapy programs, have shown to alleviate symptoms of depression and anxiety in individuals with Alzheimer's. The companionship and sensory engagement with animals contribute to a sense of joy and connection.

Drugs for Alzheimer

There are currently several medications approved by regulatory authorities for the treatment of Alzheimer's disease. These medications can help manage symptoms and slow down the progression of the disease to some extent.

1. Cholinesterase Inhibitors: Drugs such as donepezil (Aricept), rivastigmine (Exelon), and galantamine (Razadyne) work by increasing the levels of acetylcholine, a neurotransmitter that is depleted in Alzheimer's disease. These medications can help improve memory, cognition, and daily functioning in some individuals.

2. NMDA Receptor Antagonist: Memantine (Namenda) is an N-methyl-D-aspartate (NMDA) receptor antagonist that regulates glutamate, another neurotransmitter involved in learning and memory. Memantine is often used in combination with cholinesterase inhibitors to improve cognitive function and slow disease progression.

It is important to note that the effectiveness of these medications may vary among individuals, and the benefits may be modest and temporary. Additionally, these drugs may have side effects, including nausea, vomiting, dizziness, and sleep disturbances. Therefore, it is crucial to consult with a healthcare professional to assess the individual's specific situation and determine the appropriateness of medication and management options.

Other medications may also be prescribed to address specific symptoms associated with Alzheimer's disease. For example, antidepressants may be prescribed to manage mood and behavioral changes, antipsychotics may be used to manage agitation or psychosis, and sleep aids may be recommended to address sleep disturbances.

It's important to mention that researchers are actively studying and developing new drugs and treatment approaches for Alzheimer's disease. Many clinical trials are underway to investigate potential therapies aimed at slowing down or halting the progression of the disease, targeting amyloid plaques, and addressing other neurodegenerative processes associated with Alzheimer's.

While medications can provide some relief and help manage symptoms, it is important to approach Alzheimer's disease treatment holistically.

This includes implementing non-pharmacological interventions such as cognitive stimulation, physical exercise, social engagement, and a healthy lifestyle that includes a balanced diet and stress management techniques.

Monitoring Alzheimer

Monitoring individuals with Alzheimer's disease is a dynamic and vital aspect of their care, aiming to optimize their well-being, address changing needs, and provide timely interventions.

Here, we explore comprehensive strategies for monitoring Alzheimer's patients, encompassing various dimensions of their physical, cognitive, and emotional health.

Periodic assessments, including the Mini-Mental State Examination (MMSE) or Montreal Cognitive Assessment (MoCA), help track changes in memory, language, and problem-solving abilities. Daily interactions provide valuable insights into cognitive function, including memory lapses, confusion, or difficulty completing familiar tasks.

Assessing an individual's ability to perform routine tasks, such as dressing, bathing, and cooking, helps gauge functional independence. Evaluating more complex tasks like managing finances and transportation provides a broader perspective on daily functioning.

Regularly observing and documenting alterations in behavior, such as mood swings, agitation, or aggression, aids in identifying triggers and tailoring interventions. Tracking sleep quality and patterns can reveal changes that may impact overall well-being.

Regular visits to healthcare providers allow for the monitoring of physical health, identification of potential medical issues, and adjustment of medications. Verifying medication adherence is crucial for the effectiveness of Alzheimer's medications and managing coexisting conditions. Vigilance for side effects and adverse reactions necessitates open communication between caregivers, patients, and healthcare providers.

Regular assessments of the home environment help identify potential hazards, ensuring a safe living space for individuals with Alzheimer's. For those prone to wandering, implementing safety measures, such as door alarms or GPS tracking devices, is imperative.

Monitoring social interactions and engagement with loved ones helps address potential feelings of isolation and loneliness. Regular check-ins on emotional well-being, addressing any signs of anxiety or depression, contribute to a holistic approach to care.

Ensuring open lines of communication between caregivers and healthcare providers facilitates timely intervention and support.

Alzheimer Meal Plan

Day 1

Breakfast: Greek yogurt topped with a mixture of berries and granola.

Lunch: Grilled chicken breast on a bed of mixed greens, cherry tomatoes, cucumber, and a light vinaigrette dressing.

Snack: Sliced apples served with a side of almond butter.

Dinner: Baked salmon fillet served with a side of quinoa and steamed broccoli.

Smoothie: Blueberries, banana, Greek yogurt, and almond milk blended until smooth.

Day 2

Breakfast: Oatmeal topped with chopped nuts and slices of banana.

Lunch: Mixed vegetables and chickpeas stir-fried with soy sauce, served over brown rice.

Snack: Greek yogurt drizzled with honey.

Dinner: Lean ground turkey, assorted vegetables, and quinoa in a hearty broth.

Smoothie: Pineapple, mango, spinach, and coconut water blended until smooth.

Day 3

Breakfast: A thick smoothie with berries, banana, and spinach, topped with granola and shredded coconut.

Lunch: Quinoa salad with cherry tomatoes, cucumber, avocado, and a lemon-tahini dressing.

Snack: Slices of cheese served with whole grain crackers.

Dinner: Chicken seasoned with herbs, served with mashed sweet potatoes and green beans.

Smoothie: Strawberries, kiwi, Greek yogurt, and a splash of almond milk.

Day 4

Breakfast: Chia pudding made with almond milk and topped with mixed berries.

Lunch: Whole grain wrap filled with hummus, assorted vegetables, and feta cheese.

Snack: A mix of nuts, seeds, and dried fruits.

Dinner: Whole grain pasta with a tomato and lean ground turkey sauce, served with a side of steamed vegetables.

Smoothie: Mango, banana, Greek yogurt, and coconut water blended until smooth.

Day 5

Breakfast: Whole grain toast topped with sliced avocado and a poached egg.

Lunch: Grilled salmon, avocado, lettuce, and a light yogurt dressing in a whole grain wrap.

Snack: Cottage cheese paired with pineapple chunks.

Dinner: A hearty stew with lentils, various vegetables, and a flavorful broth.

Smoothie: Mixed berries, banana, spinach, and almond milk blended until smooth.

Day 6

Breakfast: Whole grain cereal with almond milk and sliced strawberries.

Lunch: Chickpeas, cherry tomatoes, cucumber, olives, and feta cheese with a lemon vinaigrette.

Snack: Fresh carrot sticks served with hummus.

Dinner: Chicken stir-fried with assorted vegetables, served over brown rice.

Smoothie: Peaches, spinach, Greek yogurt, and almond milk blended until smooth.

Day 7

Breakfast: Banana slices and peanut butter on whole grain bread.

Lunch: Quinoa, black beans, corn, tomatoes, and avocado with a lime-cilantro dressing.

Snack: Fresh berries dipped in Greek yogurt and frozen.

Dinner: Cod fillet baked with herbs, served with a side of roasted vegetables.

Smoothie: Kiwi, mixed berries, Greek yogurt, and coconut water blended until smooth.

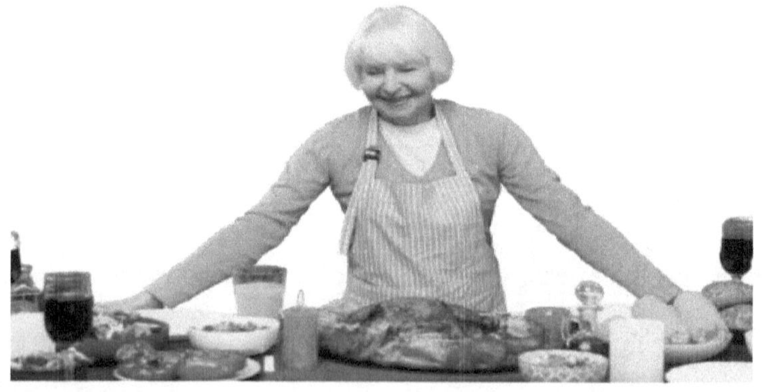

CHAPTER 4

Recipes for Alzheimer

Breakfast

1. Greek Yogurt Parfait

Ingredients

- 1 cup Greek yogurt

- 1/2 cup mixed berries (blueberries, strawberries, raspberries)

- 1/4 cup granola

- 1 tablespoon honey (optional)

Instructions

1. Arrange Greek yogurt, granola, and mixed berries in a glass or bowl.

2. Repeat the layers.

3. If desired, drizzle honey over the top.

4. Serve chilled.

2. Oatmeal with Nuts and Banana

Ingredients

- Oatmeal

- Chopped nuts (almonds, walnuts)

- Banana slices

Instructions

1. Cook oatmeal according to package instructions.

2. Top with chopped nuts and banana slices.

3. Serve warm.

3. Smoothie Bowl

Ingredients

- Mixed berries (strawberries, blueberries, raspberries)

- Banana

- Spinach leaves

- Granola

- Shredded coconut

Instructions

1. Blend a handful of mixed berries, one banana, and a handful of spinach leaves until you have a thick, smooth consistency.

2. Transfer the blended drink to a basin.

3. Top with granola and shredded coconut for added texture and flavor.

4. Enjoy with a spoon.

4. Chia Pudding with Berries

Ingredients

- Chia seeds

- Almond milk

- Mixed berries (blueberries, strawberries, raspberries)

- Honey (optional)

Instructions

1. In a bowl, mix chia seeds with almond milk. Stir well and let it sit for at least 2 hours or overnight in the refrigerator until it thickens.

2. Once the chia pudding has set, layer it with mixed berries.

3. Drizzle with honey if desired.

4. Enjoy this nutritious and satisfying breakfast.

5. Avocado Toast with Poached Egg

Ingredients

- Whole grain toast

- Ripe avocado

- Eggs

- Salt and pepper

- Optional: Red pepper flakes for spice

Instructions

1. Toast whole grain bread slices.

2. Spread a mashed, ripe avocado over the toast.

3. Poach or fry an egg and place it on top of the avocado.

4. Season with salt and pepper. Add red pepper flakes if desired.

5. Enjoy this savory and satisfying breakfast.

6. Whole Grain Cereal with Almond Milk

Ingredients

- Whole grain cereal

- Almond milk

- Sliced strawberries

Instructions

1. Pour whole grain cereal into a bowl.

2. Add almond milk.

3. Top with sliced strawberries.

4. Enjoy this quick and nutritious breakfast.

7. Peanut Butter Banana Toast

Ingredients

- Whole grain toast

- Peanut butter

- Banana slices

Instructions

1. Toast whole grain bread slices.

2. Spread peanut butter on the toast.

3. Top with banana slices.

4. Enjoy this simple and delicious peanut butter banana toast.

Lunch

1. Grilled Chicken Salad

Ingredients

- Grilled chicken breast

- Mixed greens

- Cherry tomatoes

- Cucumber

- Light vinaigrette dressing

Instructions

1. Put a platter of mixed greens together.

2. Top with grilled chicken, cherry tomatoes, and cucumber.

3. Drizzle with light vinaigrette dressing.

4. Serve.

2. Vegetable and Chickpea Stir-Fry

Ingredients

- 1 cup mixed vegetables (broccoli, bell peppers, carrots)

- 1/2 cup chickpeas (canned, drained)

- 1 tablespoon soy sauce

- 1 tablespoon olive oil

- Cooked brown rice

Instructions

1. Heat olive oil in a pan over medium heat.

2. Add mixed vegetables and stir-fry until tender.

3. Add chickpeas and soy sauce, stirring to combine.

4. Serve over cooked brown rice.

3. Quinoa Salad with Avocado

Ingredients

- Quinoa

- Cherry tomatoes, halved

- Cucumber, diced

- Avocado, diced

- Lemon-tahini dressing (mix lemon juice, tahini, olive oil, salt, and pepper)

Instructions

1. Prepare the quinoa per the instructions on the package.

2. In a bowl, combine cooked quinoa, cherry tomatoes, diced cucumber, and diced avocado.

3. Drizzle the lemon-tahini dressing over the salad and toss gently to combine.

4. Serve chilled.

4. Vegetarian Wrap

Ingredients

- Whole grain wrap

- Hummus

- Assorted vegetables (bell peppers, cucumber, carrots)

- Feta cheese, crumbled

Instructions

1. Spread a generous layer of hummus over a whole grain wrap.

2. Add a variety of colorful vegetables and crumbled feta cheese.

3. Roll the wrap tightly.

4. Slice in half and serve.

5. Salmon and Avocado Wrap

Ingredients

- Grilled salmon fillet

- Avocado slices

- Lettuce leaves

- Whole grain wrap

- Light yogurt dressing

Instructions

1. Place grilled salmon, avocado slices, and lettuce on a whole grain wrap.

2. Drizzle with a light yogurt dressing.

3. Roll the wrap tightly and cut in half.

4. Serve and relish this delicious and nutritious lunch.

6. Mediterranean Chickpea Salad

Ingredients

- Chickpeas (canned, drained)

- Cherry tomatoes, halved

- Cucumber, diced

- Kalamata olives, sliced

- Feta cheese, crumbled

- Red onion, thinly sliced

- Olive oil and lemon dressing

Instructions

1. In a bowl, combine chickpeas, cherry tomatoes, cucumber, olives, feta cheese, and red onion.

2. Drizzle with olive oil and lemon dressing.

3. Toss gently and serve this refreshing Mediterranean chickpea salad.

7. Quinoa and Black Bean Bowl

Ingredients

- Quinoa

- Black beans (canned, drained)

- Corn kernels

- Cherry tomatoes, halved

- Avocado, diced

- Lime-cilantro dressing

Instructions

1. Prepare the quinoa per the instructions on the package.

2. In a bowl, combine quinoa, black beans, corn, cherry tomatoes, and diced avocado.

3. Drizzle with lime-cilantro dressing.

4. Toss gently and serve this flavorful quinoa and black bean bowl.

Snack

1. Apple Slices with Almond Butter

Instructions

1. Slice apples.

2. Serve with a side of almond butter.

2. Greek Yogurt with Honey

Instructions

1.Pour Greek yogurt into a bowl using spoon.

2. Drizzle with honey.

3. Mix and enjoy.

3. Cheese and Whole Grain Crackers

Instructions

1. Choose your favorite type of cheese (cheddar, Swiss, or your preference).

2. Slice the cheese into bite-sized pieces.

3. Serve with whole grain crackers.

4. Enjoy this simple and satisfying snack.

4. Trail Mix

Ingredients

- Mixed nuts (almonds, walnuts, cashews)

- Dried fruits (apricots, raisins, cranberries)

- Dark chocolate chips

Instructions

1. Mix together your favorite nuts, dried fruits, and dark chocolate chips.

2. Portion out into snack-sized servings.

3. Enjoy this energy-boosting trail mix.

5. Cottage Cheese with Pineapple

Instructions

1. Pour cottage cheese into a bowl using a spoon.

2. Add chunks of fresh pineapple.

3. Mix and savor this protein-rich and refreshing snack.

6. Carrot Sticks with Hummus

Instructions

1. Wash and cut fresh carrot sticks.

2. Dip in hummus.

3. Enjoy this crunchy and satisfying snack.

7. Yogurt-Covered Berries

Ingredients

- Fresh berries (strawberries, blueberries, raspberries)

- Greek yogurt

Instructions

1. Dip fresh berries into Greek yogurt, covering them partially.

2. Place on a tray lined with parchment paper.

3. Freeze until the yogurt is set.

4. Enjoy these refreshing yogurt-covered berries as a cool snack.

Dinner

1. Baked Salmon with Quinoa

Ingredients

- Baked salmon fillet

- Cooked quinoa

- Steamed broccoli

Instructions

1. Serve baked salmon on a bed of cooked quinoa.

2. Add steamed broccoli on the side.

3. Enjoy.

2. Turkey and Vegetable Soup

Ingredients

- Lean ground turkey

- Assorted vegetables (carrots, celery, onions)

- Quinoa

- Chicken or vegetable broth

Instructions

1. Brown ground turkey in a pot.

2. Add chopped vegetables, quinoa, and broth.

3. Simmer until vegetables are tender.

4. Serve hot.

3. Pour into a glass and enjoy.

3. Baked Herb Chicken with Sweet Potato Mash

Ingredients

- Chicken breasts, boneless and skinless

- Assorted herbs (rosemary, thyme)

- Sweet potatoes, peeled and cubed

- Olive oil

- Salt and pepper

- Steamed green beans

Instructions

1. Turn the oven on to 375°F (190°C).

2. Rub chicken breasts with a mixture of olive oil, chopped rosemary, thyme, salt, and pepper.

3. Place the chicken on a baking sheet and bake until fully cooked.

4. Boil sweet potatoes until tender, then mash with a touch of olive oil, salt, and pepper.

5. Serve the baked herb chicken on a bed of sweet potato mash with steamed green beans on the side.

4. Pasta with Tomato and Turkey Sauce

Ingredients

- Whole grain pasta

- Lean ground turkey

- Tomato sauce

- Garlic, minced

- Olive oil

- Spinach leaves

Instructions

1. Cook whole grain pasta according to package instructions.

2. In a pan, sauté minced garlic in olive oil.

3. Add ground turkey and cook until browned.

4. Pour in tomato sauce and simmer.

5. Stir in fresh spinach leaves until wilted.

6. Over the cooked pasta, serve the sauce.

5. Vegetable and Lentil Stew

Ingredients

- Green or brown lentils

- Assorted vegetables (carrots, celery, potatoes)

- Onion, chopped

- Garlic, minced

- Vegetable broth

- Tomato paste

- Herbs (rosemary, thyme)

- Salt and pepper

Instructions

1. Rinse lentils and set aside.

2. In a pot, sauté chopped onions and minced garlic until fragrant.

3. Add lentils, assorted vegetables, vegetable broth, tomato paste, herbs, salt, and pepper.

4. Simmer until lentils and vegetables are tender.

5. Serve this hearty and nutritious vegetable and lentil stew.

6. Chicken Stir-Fry with Brown Rice

Ingredients

- Chicken breast, thinly sliced

- Mixed vegetables (broccoli, bell peppers, snap peas)

- Soy sauce

- Olive oil

- Brown rice, cooked

Instructions

1. In a wok or pan, heat olive oil.

2. Add thinly sliced chicken and stir-fry until browned.

3. Add mixed vegetables and soy sauce, continue stir-frying until vegetables are tender.

4. Serve over cooked brown rice.

7. Baked Cod with Roasted Vegetables

Ingredients

- Cod fillet

- Olive oil

- Lemon juice

- Assorted vegetables (zucchini, bell peppers, cherry tomatoes)

- Herbs (rosemary, thyme)

- Salt and pepper

Instructions

1. Turn the oven on to 400°F (200°C).

2. Place cod fillet on a baking sheet.

3. Add a lemon juice and olive oil drizzle. Season with herbs, salt, and pepper.

4. Surround the cod with assorted vegetables.

5. Bake until the cod is cooked through and the vegetables are tender.

6. Serve this baked cod with roasted vegetables.

Smoothies

1. Blueberry Banana Smoothie

Ingredients

- 1 cup blueberries

- 1 banana

- 1/2 cup Greek yogurt

- 1/2 cup almond milk

- Ice cubes (optional)

Instructions

1. Blend blueberries, banana, Greek yogurt, and almond milk until smooth.

2. Add ice cubes and blend again if desired.

3. Pour into a glass and serve immediately.

2. Green Tropical Smoothie

Ingredients

- 1 cup pineapple chunks

- 1/2 cup mango chunks

- Handful of spinach leaves

- 1/2 cup coconut water

- Ice cubes

Instructions

1. Blend pineapple, mango, spinach, and coconut water until smooth.

2. Add ice cubes and blend again.

3. Strawberry Kiwi Smoothie

Ingredients

- Strawberries

- Kiwi

- Greek yogurt

- Almond milk

Instructions:

1. Blend strawberries, peeled kiwi, Greek yogurt, and almond milk until smooth.

2. Adjust the consistency by adding more almond milk if needed.

3. Pour into a glass and enjoy this refreshing smoothie.

4. Mango Banana Smoothie

Ingredients

- Mango

- Banana

- Greek yogurt

- Coconut water

Instructions

1. Blend mango, banana, Greek yogurt, and coconut water until smooth.

2. Adjust the consistency by adding more coconut water if needed.

3. Pour into a glass and enjoy this tropical-inspired smoothie.

5. Mixed Berry Smoothie

Ingredients

- Mixed berries (strawberries, blueberries, raspberries)

- Banana

- Spinach leaves

- Almond milk

Instructions

1. Blend mixed berries, banana, spinach, and almond milk until smooth.

2. Adjust the consistency with more almond milk if needed.

3. Pour into a glass and enjoy this antioxidant-rich smoothie.

6. Peach and Spinach Smoothie

Ingredients

- Peaches (fresh or frozen)

- Spinach leaves

- Greek yogurt

- Almond milk

Instructions

1. Blend peaches, spinach, Greek yogurt, and almond milk until smooth.

2. Adjust the consistency with more almond milk if needed.

3. Pour into a glass and enjoy this nutritious peach and spinach smoothie.

7. Kiwi Berry Smoothie

Ingredients

- Kiwi

- Mixed berries (strawberries, blueberries, raspberries)

- Greek yogurt

- Coconut water

Instructions

1. Blend peeled kiwi, mixed berries, Greek yogurt, and coconut water until smooth.

2. If necessary, adjust the consistency by adding extra almond milk.

3. Transfer to a glass and savor this cool smoothie.

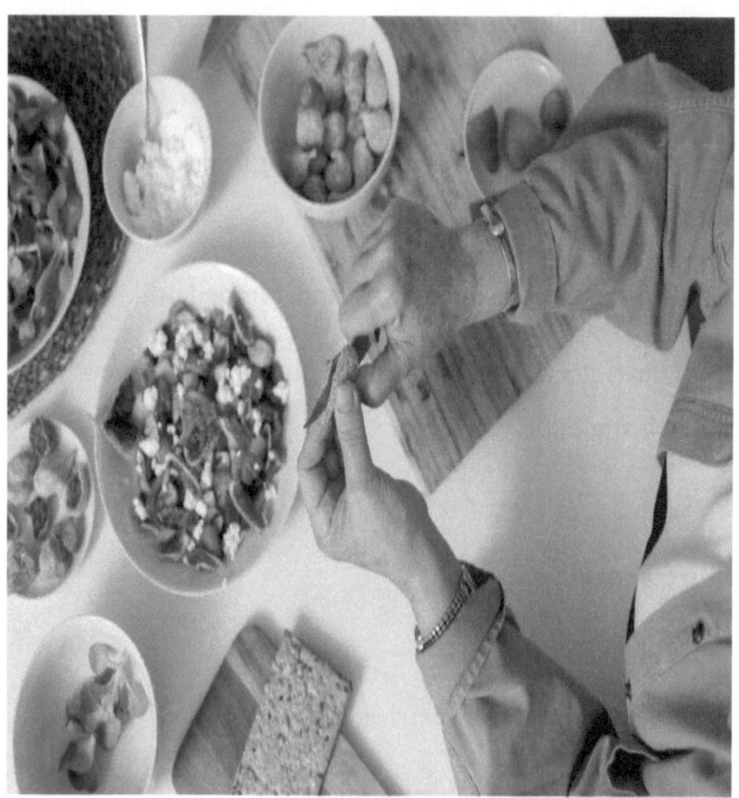

Conclusion

In conclusion, this Alzheimer Recipe Cookbook is designed with a deep commitment to promoting the well-being of individuals living with Alzheimer's disease. Each recipe has been thoughtfully crafted to not only cater to the nutritional needs of those on the Alzheimer's journey but also to provide a palate of flavors that can bring joy and satisfaction to the dining experience.

Recognizing the challenges that individuals with Alzheimer's face, the cookbook emphasizes simplicity in preparation while maintaining a focus on nutrient-dense ingredients. The recipes are diverse, offering a variety of options for breakfast, lunch, dinner, snacks, and smoothies, ensuring a balanced and enjoyable approach to nutrition.

The underlying philosophy of this cookbook extends beyond the kitchen; it embraces the idea that food is not only sustenance but a source of comfort, connection, and joy. It acknowledges the role that well-planned, nutritious meals play in supporting cognitive health and overall quality of life for those navigating the complexities of Alzheimer's.

As we conclude this epicurean voyage, it is our hope that these recipes not only inspire delicious and healthful meals but also contribute to a positive and dignified dining experience. May this cookbook serve as a guide for caregivers, families, and individuals alike, fostering a deeper understanding of the significance of nutrition and the joy that can be found in sharing a thoughtfully prepared meal. Together, let us continue to create moments of nourishment, connection, and well-being for those touched by Alzheimer's.